VALIANT DOCTORS

IN THE

FRONTIER WEST

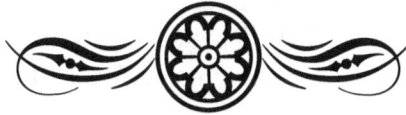

DOROTHY AUDREY SIMPSON, ED. D.

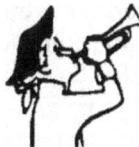

HERITAGE BOOKS
2020

HERITAGE BOOKS

AN IMPRINT OF HERITAGE BOOKS, INC.

Books, CDs, and more—Worldwide

For our listing of thousands of titles see our website
at
www.HeritageBooks.com

Published 2020 by
HERITAGE BOOKS, INC.
Publishing Division
5810 Ruatan Street
Berwyn Heights, Md. 20740

Heritage Books by the author:

*From Pajarito to Lungchow: Memoirs of
Photographic Reconnaissance Pilot Stanley A. Hardin*

Quatie Ross: First Lady of the Cherokee Nation

Valiant Doctors in the Frontier West

International Standard Book Number
Paperbound: 978-0-7884-5801-9

To my grandchildren

TABLE OF CONTENTS

CHAPTER

Page

CHAPTER 1

Doctors in New Spain

Smallpox caused the deaths of countless victims at the time of the exploration of the New World. About 400,000 Europeans died each year of smallpox in the Eighteenth Century. Most people became infected at some time during their lifetimes. A good number of those survived, although they probably carried the scars to show it.

In the late 1700's, an English physician, Dr. Edward Jenner, developed a smallpox vaccine which he hoped would prevent the disease. It proved to be successful. In 1799, an American physician, Dr. Valentine Seaman, administered the first smallpox vaccine in the United States. His first child had died of smallpox in 1795. After that he gave his remaining children a smallpox vaccination, using the serum acquired from Dr. Jenner.

According to Richard Dunlop in *Doctors of the American Frontier*, Francisco Xavier de Balmis, in 1803, brought a cargo of children who were to form a living chain of vaccine carriers to the New World. When the ship landed in Mexico with its chain of living virus, Dr. Xavier de Balmis set about vaccinating the population. On

April 8, 1806, the life-saving virus reached Texas, the remote frontier of the Spanish Empire. When adults saw that the children who had been vaccinated were disease free, they accepted the vaccination.

In 1792, the first Spanish doctor settled in Santa Fe. He was Dr. Cristóval María Larrañaga. Born in Spain, Larrañaga immigrated to Mexico and then to what is now northern New Mexico. He married María Gertrudiz Mestas. They had seven sons and two daughters. In 1804 Larrañaga received a shipment of cowpox scabs from Mexico City. He travelled north to Chihuahua City with children to pass the smallpox vaccination from person to person, just as Dr. Xavier de Balmis had done a year earlier. Larrañaga continued his trip north until he reached Taos, New Mexico. His records show he vaccinated 3,610 people. People in the area had been struggling against smallpox since the early 1780s. In 1781 smallpox killed 5,000 people, perhaps more than a quarter of the population of what is now New Mexico. According to Fray Angélico Chávez, in 1809 Dr. Larrañaga vaccinated until he ran out of the vaccine. In 1810, he was recorded as vaccinating 124 children up to age six. As the only trained physician in the entire territory, he was responsible for the care of more than forty thousand people. It was said that he was exhausted, but he carried on as long as possible. He was thought of by many as a pioneer hero.

The first doctors in the West came to the New World with the Spanish explorers. In 1535, Alvar Núñez Cabeza de Vaca explored the New World and brought his surgeon with him. A physician also accompanied Francisco Vásquez de Coronado on his explorations from 1536 to 1540. As Coronado searched for the fabled Seven Cities of Gold, some of the Native Americans fought against the newcomers. Coronado was wounded with a poisoned arrow. Indians had used such arrows for many years. Coronado's physician treated the wound with quince juice. Coronado recovered. (Note that the term "Native American" and "Indian" are used interchangeably since much of the literature uses both terms.)

There were many other times that a doctor saved a life in the New World, as the Spaniards--and later other groups--infiltrated the world of the Native Americans. In 1810, freedom was won from the Spanish king, and the people living in New Spain came under the rule of Mexico. In 1821, the independent Mexicans, who had put an end to the Spanish aversion to outsiders, began to welcome newcomers. That meant that Americans could cross the Mexican border freely into what is now Texas, Arizona, New Mexico and California.

William Bucknell began using the Santa Fe Trail in 1821. Starting in Franklin, Missouri, the Santa Fe Trail went through Kansas, Oklahoma, Colorado and finally to Santa Fe, New Mexico. The Trail witnessed a furious heyday between 1830 and 1848 as a trade route linking Santa Fe, New Mexico and Los Angeles, California.

The community which became known as Las Vegas, New Mexico grew as trade on the Santa Fe Trail became more and more prolific. Las Vegas was one of the main stopping places on the Trail. More Americans began to arrive in the area, and with them, more physicians came to the west.

In 1827, Dr. David Waldo was the first doctor from the United States of America to settle in what would become known as New Mexico Territory--which then belonged to Mexico. He settled in Santa Fe and practiced medicine there and in the surrounding areas.

A year later, another doctor from the east settled in that area.

His name was Dr. Henry Connelly, an early trader on the Santa Fe Trail. Connelly was the first doctor to settle in Las Vegas, New Mexico in 1828. Connelly was married twice, first while residing in Chihuahua, and he had a son named Peter. Henry's wife died a few years later. After some time, Henry Connelly married Dolores Perea, the widow of Mariano Chavez, the father of J. Francisco Chavez who helped in the founding of the public school system in New Mexico.

Dr. Connelly opened the Chihuahua Trail in 1828. He had mercantile establishments expanding from Las Vegas to Chihuahua, Mexico. At that time Las Vegas was the largest town in the Territory. He had a store in Las Vegas and had a thriving business there in 1846 when General Stephen W. Kearny made his famous proclamation, making New Mexico a part of the United States of America. Connelly's place of business in Las Vegas was on the west side of the Plaza, at the south intersection of the Plaza and North National Street. He sold the place in 1863.

Dr. Connelly was appointed Governor of New Mexico Territory by President Abraham Lincoln. On March 4, 1862, before the fall of Santa Fe into Confederate General Henry H. Sibley's hands,

Connelly moved the seat of government of the Territory to Las Vegas. Thus, Las Vegas became the Capital of New Mexico Territory and remained so until after the Battle of Glorieta and until after the Confederates had been driven south of Albuquerque, a period of about six weeks. Thereafter, Santa Fe was again the capital. Connelly died in July of 1866 in Santa Fe.

In 1835 settlers found the area now known as Las Vegas to be a good place for their homes and their livestock. A village was built around a plaza. According to Milton W. Callon in *Las Vegas, New Mexico...The Town That Wouldn't Gamble*, the Cabeza de Baca family moved to the Las Vegas area before 1823. They brought their excellent herd of horses and mules--six hundred in all.

Another of the early doctors to travel over the Santa Fe Trail was Dr. Josiah Gregg. In 1831, he came over the Trail and recorded his observations in journals. He wrote *Commerce of the Prairies.* Unfortunately, he had tuberculosis and was too ill to practice medicine. However, he found the climate of the Southwest to be very good. He recommended the area to sufferers, believing that they might thrive if they came to the Southwest where the climate was warm, sunny, and dry. For many years the area of New Mexico attracted tuberculosis patients in hopes of finding relief from the ravages of that disease.

They came by ship, then by wagon or by horseback: those brave pioneers looking for life in the New World. The doctors came with them seeking a salubrious climate, seeking a richer life, seeking to serve those courageous souls whose homes in Europe were to be exchanged for the unknown in the New World. The Spanish *padres* (priests) hoped to show the Native Americans the way of salvation. The doctors came with them, hoping to show them all the way of health.

REFERENCES

Beimer, Dorothy Simpson, "Pioneer Physicians in Las Vegas, New Mexico: 1880-1911," unpublished manuscript, 1975, in Donnelly Library, New Mexico Highlands University, Las Vegas, New Mexico.

Chávez, Fray Angélico *Origins of New Mexico Families: A Genealogy of the Spanish Colonial Period*. Albuquerque, New Mexico: Museum of New Mexico Press, 1992

Milton W. Callon. *Las Vegas, New Mexico...The Town that Wouldn't Gamble*. Las Vegas, New Mexico: The Las Vegas Publishing Co, Inc., 1962, pp. 4-8

Richard Dunlop. "Spanish Doctors," in *Doctors of the American Frontier*. New York: Ballantine Books, 1965, pp. 51-53.

Lucas, William J. *Why Fort Union?* unpublished manuscript, Las Vegas, New Mexico, 1929, in Donnelly Library, New Mexico Highlands University, Las Vegas, New Mexico.

Thatcher, Harold F., "Frontier Southwest Americans," unpublished manuscript, Las Vegas, New Mexico, 1978.

CHAPTER 2

Wagon Train Doctors

There were many reasons doctors came in the early days of this country to settle in the west. Two well-known routes were the Santa Fe Trail and the Oregon Trail. People who traveled the Santa Fe Trail were, for the most part, individual male traders who continued to travel back and forth between Santa Fe and the United States to buy and sell American factory goods. The people who traveled on the Oregon Trail in the mid-1800's were more likely to be families wanting to settle in Oregon. However, both trails attracted those seeking riches, especially when it was learned that gold had been discovered in one place or another.

From the mid-1830's, particularly through the years 1846-1869, the Oregon Trail was used by about 400,000 travelers. The Oregon Trail started in Missouri, then crossed Kansas, Nebraska, Wyoming, Idaho, and finally ended in Oregon. The Oregon Trail was 2,170 miles across the country, starting from Independence, Missouri and ending in Oregon City, Oregon. Before leaving Independence, Missouri, in preparing for the trip, the people would elect a wagon master and hire veteran frontiersmen to guide them.

In 1844, there were 1,475 emigrants bound for Oregon. In 1845 there were 2,400 emigrants. With the 1849 gold rush, more travelers chose California as their final destination, but Oregon still had many wanting to settle there. Between 1841 and 1866, about 350,000 people went over the Oregon Trail. Emigrants to California and Oregon had to cover about 2,000 miles between one winter and the next. Pioneers traveling in covered wagons hoped to reach their destinations before the first snowfall in the high mountain passes. If they made good time, starting in April, they might reach their destination by November.

After travel along the Sweetwater River in Wyoming, the pioneers came to Independence Rock. They traveled through the South Pass into the Wind River Mountains in Wyoming. They went to Pacific Springs, Wyoming and moved on to Fort Bridger. They traveled on to Soda Springs, Idaho and finally arrived at Fort Hall, a supply depot operated by the Hudson's Bay Company in Oregon Territory. It was at Fort Hall, 55 miles beyond Soda Springs, that the wagons split up, with one part going on to California and the other on to Oregon.

Some of the doctors traveled with the Spanish explorers or came on the Santa Fe Trail, as mentioned previously. Some came to trade. Some came to find a healthful climate. Some wanted a place to retire away from the big cities. Some came with the forts, such as Fort Union, 26 miles northwest of Las Vegas, New Mexico. Some in military service later chose private practice. Some came with the opening of the railroad as populations exploded and businesses created jobs. There were mining town doctors who served the population of miners and trappers, men who opened up the west along with farmers and ranchers. There were cowboy doctors who lived near ranches or cow-shipping towns and cared for the ranchers and cowboys. Some even accompanied the cowboys on their trail drives as the cattle were taken to market many miles away. There were frontier-town doctors who drove horses and buggies to make house calls in the remote country areas where their patients lived outside of the settlements. There were country doctors of all kinds, those who traveled by horseback, by horse and buggy, by covered wagon or, later, by railroad.

For whatever reason, people came over the Santa Fe and Oregon Trails on their way west, traveling in canvas covered wagons known as prairie schooners or covered wagons. The wagons had 10 by 3 1/2 foot bodies. The Conestoga wagon could transport up to six tons of cargo under good conditions, pulled by horses, mules or oxen. The heavier the wagon, however, the more likely it would bog down in mud or cause the team to break down with fatigue. Travelers were advised to keep their wagons weighing less than 1 1/2 tons, fully loaded. A few people would actually take two wagons in order to have enough supplies for the trip. But it cost about a hundred dollars for each loaded wagon. If the oxen or mules became exhausted or if the trail was too hazardous for a heavy wagon, the loads would have to be lightened. The trails were often littered with many items that had to be left behind, such things as stoves, trunks of clothes, oak bureaus, cooking pots, tables, and so on.

Including its tongue, the average Conestoga wagon was 18 feet long, 11 feet high and 4 feet in width. Their covers were made of canvas or waterproofed sheeting. Hickory bows supported the cloth tops. The rear wheels of a wagon were 5 or 6 feet in diameter, but the front wheels were 4 feet in diameter or less to protect the body of the wagon on sharp turns. The wheels were made of iron and wooden rims. Unfortunately, the rims and spokes would sometimes crack and split, especially if they became too dry.

Isaac Jones Wistar was a lawyer in Philadelphia. He heard about gold in California and went by wagon train in 1849 to become a miner in the gold fields. On the way to California, he kept a journal. He wrote that someone was ill and he hoped it was not smallpox. He feared the illness would cause a significant delay. Jones said that to empty a wagon and take the sick man back to Independence, Missouri would cause delay that might have serious results should the west-bound people arrive at the Sierra too late to cross for the year. The sick man grew worse. The wagon train doctor insisted that the pioneers halt their wagons. In spite of his efforts, the doctor was unable to save his patient. Although the sick man did not recover, he was surrounded by friends who allowed him to die in peace.

Dr. John Powell traveled on the Oregon Trail in 1852 and cared for the sick of his train. He rode fifty miles out of the way to care for patients traveling with other wagon trains. He delivered babies and fought typhoid and cholera.

Dr. C. M. Clark accompanied a wagon train in 1860 in the Pike's Peak gold rush. Typhoid fever, scurvy, smallpox, cholera, tuberculosis, and wounds inflicted by Indians all took their toll. Clark wrote that sickness often visited the emigrant. He identified the prevailing diseases as bilious fever, which often assumed a typhoid character; pleurisy; pneumonia; and scurvy; and there were other ailments due to exposure to weather, improper or insufficient food, and over-exertion. Many suffered from diarrhea and dysentery.

Dr. Elijah White was captain of the wagon train as well as wagon train doctor when he led a train of 100 settlers to Oregon in 1842. Dr. Justin Millard, too, led a party, taking them safely to the northwest in 1852.

Dr. Thomas Flint of Maine drove 2,000 sheep and numerous horses, cows and oxen from Illinois to California, in spite of hostile Indians. He stood off the attacks of bears and wolves, and he took his people across the Mohave Desert. He settled down to practice at San Juan Bautista in California.

According to Bob Brooke in "Wagon Tracks West," in the

August, 1993 issue of *Wild West*, Dr. Marcus Whitman, a Protestant missionary and physician, joined a wagon train after his return west following a trip east. He was called "that good angel" of the emigrants. They felt they were indebted to him for getting them through their journey. Dr. Whitman and his nephew, Perrin Whitman, were excellent guides as the wagons crossed the rough terrain. Dr. Whitman's medical skill was of tremendous worth to the people who fell ill. All too many people died along to trail. However, when babies were born, the pioneers were hopeful. Dr. Whitman's advice to the travelers was, "Keep moving."

In 1843 a wagon train bound for Oregon chose Peter Burnett as captain and Jesse Applegate as a leader. Mountain man John Gant was the chief guide as far as Fort Hall. That wagon train included nearly 1,000 people and more than 200 wagons, as well as 700 oxen and nearly 800 cattle.

According to Bob Brooke in his *Wild West* article, each evening the wagons were parked in a circle. The rear wagon was connected with the wagon in front by its tongue and ox chains. The circled wagons served as a corral for livestock. The chains were strong enough to keep the oxen from breaking out. The circle also served as a good barricade should Indians attack. There were usually guards on duty all night. Indian war parties seldom attacked a circle of wagons, however, knowing there would be heavy casualties among them. The new day usually started when sentinels fired their rifles at four o'clock in the morning. The wagon train was ready to move by seven o'clock.

In Season 1, Episode 19 of "Wagon Train," Charles Bickford plays the title in role "The Daniel Barrister Story." The TV show stars Ward Bond as Major Seth Adams, Wagon Master, with Scout Flint McCullough played by Robert Horton. Directed by Richard Bartlett, the story begins when a woman is thrown from a wagon, badly injured, but her husband abhors doctors. McCullough finds Dr. Peter H. Culver, played by Roger Smith, in a nearby town. Culver has been fighting a smallpox epidemic but goes to the wagon train and convinces Barrister to allow him to treat the woman, and she recovers.

In December of 1956, a Walt Disney film entitled "Westward Ho the Wagons!" was released to theatres by Buena Vista Distribution Company. It starred Kathleen Crowley, Jeff York, and the popular

Fess Parker (who also played Davy Crocket and Daniel Boone in other productions.) Parker played the role of the wagon train's doctor who was going west with the pioneers. In an encounter with Native Americans, the doctor saves the life of an Indian boy and gains the respect of the tribe, giving them safe passage through the land. This movie portrayed the importance of attaining the good will of the Native Americans and the significant role a doctor could play to that end. The movie was based on a novel by Mary Jane Carr, *Children of the Covered Wagon.*

The 1959 movie, "The Horse Soldiers," starred John Wayne, Constance Towers, and William Holden as an Army doctor. The crude surgery of that time depicted a doctor's attempt to save the lives of the wounded. While movies may portray life in a Hollywood reality, the true-to-life doctors often faced similar situations.

Not only did they often work under stressful situations, but often their patients were poor people who could not pay. Doctors treated the poor as well as the affluent patients with equal care. The doctor was obligated to provide for their medicines and their various therapies. Some of the frontier doctors made a living by doing other things when the practice of medicine was not very lucrative. Numerous early day doctors established businesses in addition to their private practices. It was previously mentioned that Dr. Josiah Gregg was a successful businessman, as was Dr. Henry Connelly.

For whatever reasons they moved west, men and women of valor faced unknown dangers. Travel was slow and laborious over the rough trails. Often survival depended on the livestock. That meant having sufficient food and water not only for themselves but for their animals. A broken wagon wheel, a sudden storm, a river crossing, a deep canyon, a mountain trail, hostile enemy attacks, and the ever-present danger of illness, injury or disease--all these presented challenges as the pioneers headed west. If the wagon train was lucky enough to have a doctor "on board" that was a definite plus.

Wagons were often so filled with supplies that there was little room for travelers to stretch out and sleep in a wagon. More often than not, night time rest was taken under a wagon where wind, rain, hail, or sand storms could disturb a good night's sleep. Oxen and horses and mules toiled westward over the trails from sunrise into the setting sun when a restful night under the stars meant a few more miles toward a destination--and a destiny.

A good description of life on the wagon train--and the key role played by physicians at that time--was given by author Laura H. Shepherd Lewis, Ph.D. in her book *My Name is Mary Elizabeth: Westward Through the Eyes of a Child.* Lewis' books is based on a true account written in a journal by Mary Elizabeth who left her home in St. Louis, Missouri to travel over the Oregon Trail with her parents, John and Mary Eloise, and her little brother Josiah (Josh.) They hoped to settle on farm land in Oregon. Although Mary Elizabeth was only eleven years of age, she was a very good writer. The journal was written on penny tablets, on both sides of the page, with a soft leaded pencil. Spelling was phonetic for the most part. It was mostly printed, with some cursive writing throughout. Mary Elizabeth described many events, including some frightening ones. The journal was given by Mary Elizabeth to Laura Lewis' grandfather, Dr. John C. Shepherd, M.D. He passed it on to his granddaughter Laura who wrote the book about the wagon train based on the journal.

The journal of Mary Elizabeth gives details about the trip itself, the items they took with them in the wagon; terrain they crossed; the rivers they forded; the care of the livestock; the food they prepared; and even the dangers of other humans, not just hostile Native Americans. Through Missouri and Kansas, especially, there were gangs of white marauders. If those thieves found a wagon alone, or just a few wagons, they would attack. They would kill everyone in the wagons and take everything of value.

For a period of time, Mary Elizabeth and her parents (John and Mary Eloise) did travel alone. The people of the wagon train they started out with urged the family to leave them because of fear of tuberculosis, for Mary Elizabeth's mother was in the last stages of the disease when they started the trip. The woman knew she was dying, but she wanted to travel west. She urged her daughter to keep a journal about the trip. The family made the sick woman as comfortable as they could. They made room for her to sleep in the wagon while they slept outside under the wagon. They gave her the best care possible. But the danger to a single wagon was a constant worry.

One day John went to move the mules to a new grass site, leaving Mary Eloise propped against a tree on pillows. Suddenly three white men came riding up with their guns at the ready. Josh (Mary Elizabeth's little brother) and Mary Elizabeth were hiding inside the wagon, as they had been taught to do if they sensed danger.

One of the men began to make comments about a beautiful woman all alone and what he intended for them to do before they took everything of value from the wagon. But Mary Eloise was prepared, in spite of her illness. She raised her gun and pointed it at the threatening man. The outlaw laughed, thinking the woman was too frail to actually shoot him. She did shoot. He died instantly. At the same time, Mary Elizabeth, whose father had taught her to shoot, looked out from the wagon, aimed her rifle at the second man, and pulled the trigger. He fell onto his horse's neck and rode off with the terrorized third man.

When John returned, he learned what had happened. He knew that Mary Elizabeth was upset about shooting a man. He explained to his daughter that some men were evil and that they had to be fought against. He told her that he was proud of her, for she had fought evil and helped save their lives. Naturally, John was also proud of his wife for defending herself.

Soon thereafter Mary Eloise succumbed to the deadly disease that they called "lung fever." Mary Elizabeth and Josh helped their father bury Mary Eloise along the trail. Then they returned to re-join the wagon train they had left. The wagons were stationed outside of a small Nebraska town.

Unfortunately, smallpox had decimated the wagon train, which was one of the last to cross over the Trail and was also one of the largest wagon trains, in terms of numbers, ever to follow the Oregon Trail. Those numbers dwindled as each wagon lost at least one person to smallpox. Some entire families were wiped out.

Mary Elizabeth's little brother, Josiah, played with some boys who had been exposed to smallpox. In fact, they were coming down with the disease. Before long, Josh got sick and then died. Mary Elizabeth and her father buried the boy in a grave next to his mother's. Soon thereafter, John got smallpox and he also died.

Mary Elizabeth describes the compassionate doctor (Dr. John C. Shepherd) who came twice a day from the near-by Nebraska community to care for those stricken with smallpox in the wagon train, which was located well outside of the town. The wagon master had died of the disease and there were very few people left to care for the sick. The doctor found a few people who had already survived smallpox in the past to help care for the stricken.

Mary Elizabeth's journal describes the sick and dying, as well as the efforts of all who tried to help them. So many died that there were not enough men to keep up with the job of digging graves to bury the dead. If an entire family died, men burned the entire wagon with the bodies inside. Quite a few wagons were burned, including that of the wagon master whose death left the people without a leader. Unfortunately, he was the only person with a list of all the people on the wagon train, along with the addresses of their relatives. Hence, after the epidemic had ended, there was no way to notify relatives that their loved ones had died along the trail.

Mary Elizabeth escaped smallpox, but she was an orphan. Dr. Shepherd had worked tirelessly during the epidemic, knowing the disease had no cure, but doing his best to pull his patients through. The concerned doctor arranged for a couple on the wagon train to adopt Mary Elizabeth. As she said good-by to the kind doctor, Mary Elizabeth gave him the journal she had written all along the way.

Then she proceeded on to Oregon with her new family and the survivors of the epidemic under a new wagon master.

Dr. John C. Shepherd lived in a small southeastern Nebraska river town called Rulo, on the west bank of the Missouri River. The journal he was given finally fell into the hands of Dr. Shepherd's granddaughter. Based on Mary Elizabeth's journal, Dr. Laura H. Shepherd Lewis wrote the book about the young girl's journey and her description of how Dr. Shepherd had helped during the smallpox epidemic.

Those who survived the disease continued on their trip to Oregon. A very few, like Mary Elizabeth, escaped it altogether. She never forgot the kindness of Dr. Shepherd, nor did the survivors of the wagon train on the trail to Oregon.

REFERENCES

Beimer, Dorothy Simpson, "Pioneer Physicians in Las Vegas, New Mexico: 1880-1911," unpublished manuscript, 1975, in Donnelly Library, New Mexico Highlands University, Las Vegas, New Mexico.

Brooke Bob. "Wagon Tracks West," *Wild West*, August, 1993, pp. 42- 51.

Lewis, Laura H. Shepherd. *My Name is Mary Elizabeth: Westward Through the Eyes of a Child*. X-libris Corporation, 2004.

Simpson, Dorothy Audrey. *Audrey of the Mountains: The Story of a Twentieth Century Pioneer Woman*. Santa Fe: Sunstone Press, 2008.

CHAPTER 3

Doctors at Forts

The American west had many forts. A fortification was a military construction of buildings designed for the defense of territories in warfare--and was also used to solidify rule in a region during peacetime. When Native Americans posed a threat to the European immigrants, forts were established. When the Civil War required soldiers to be housed and trained, the forts were essential. They served to protect civilians, as well. There were, at one time, 21 forts just in the Territory of New Mexico alone. For instance, there was Fort Wingate, 11 miles east of Gallup; Fort Marcy, just north and east of Santa Fe; Fort Sumner, about five miles southeast of the town of Fort Sumner; Fort Stanton, nine miles west of Lincoln; and Fort Union, seven miles northwest of Watrous. Kansas had the most forts, around 77 in all, including Fort Dodge, Fort Hays, Fort Leavenworth, Fort McKean and Fort Riley, to name a few. Texas had 43 forts, such as Fort Clark, Fort Crockett, Fort Gates, Fort Hood, Fort Sam Houston, and Fort Lancaster. A complete list of forts can be found in Wikipedia's "Forts in the American Old West" on the internet.

The first hospital west of the Mississippi River was at Fort Union, constructed in 1851 just twenty-six miles northeast of Las Vegas, the largest town in New Mexico Territory at the time. In the spring of 1851, the first fort was constructed. Soldiers stationed at Fort Union went on Indian campaigns, furnished escorts for travelers and the postal service, sometimes rescued captured citizens. The fort had a huge parade ground, surrounded by adobe officers' quarters, barracks, offices, warehouses, stables, a jail and chapel. At Fort Union, the 36-bed hospital served both soldiers and civilians. During the Civil War, General Edward Canby moved the fort a mile north and it was enlarged and improved.

According to the article by Audrey Simpson, "The Fort that Won the West" published in December, 1950 *New Mexico Magazine*, five raiding tribes--the Utahs, Kiowas, Navajos, Apaches, and Comanches--caused property loss that was estimated in official records at $114,500 during the 1849-1850 period. The Native Americans swooped down upon settlements, wagon trains and ranches, killing, plundering, kidnapping and driving off stock. Fort Marcy was unable to protect the traders' slow freight wagons over the long miles from St. Louis, Missouri. Fort Union housed one thousand and more troops and had stable facilities with a capacity of a thousand head of stock. The Sutler's store did a daily average of $3,000 business. Fort Union remained an important part of New Mexico Territory until after the coming of the telegraph and the railroad--until 1891.

Fort Union protected the Santa Fe Trail. It was one fort that did not fall to the Confederate Army and so perhaps saved the whole west from the Confederates, may have even changed the course of the Civil War, according to Audrey Simpson's article, "The Fort that Won the West."

There were good facilities at Fort Union, so several doctors were attracted there. When they left the military service, a number of them chose to stay in New Mexico. For instance, **Dr. C. C. Gordon** served at Fort Union and later moved to Las Vegas where he had a private practice and joined the Las Vegas Medical Society which was organized in 1882.

Dr. E. R. Squibb (Edward Robinson Squibb) came to Las Vegas after leaving Fort Union. He arrived in New Mexico Territory in the early 1850's at Fort Union with the Army and then later established himself in Las Vegas. His side line was a manufacturing chemist and he produced the first chloroform for use in the west. Later he was a leading manufacturer of pharmaceuticals and founded E. R. Squibb & Sons, which eventually became part of the modern pharmaceutical giant Bristol-Meyers. Dr. Squibb's sons were Edward H. Squibb and Charles F. Squibb. This outstanding man, Dr. E. R. Squibb, went from Fort Union to Las Vegas because he liked New Mexico and found it conducive to his work.

Another of the medical men to stay in New Mexico after leaving Fort Union was Dr. John H. Shout. He had an interesting military background. Born in New York, John Shout graduated from a college in Vermont, practiced in Iowa, and was attracted west by gold in Colorado. He moved to Taos, New Mexico Territory in 1859 or 1860. In 1862, he received the appointment of regimental surgeon in Kit Carson's regiment, First New Mexico Volunteers, and was stationed at Fort Union.

In 1865, Dr. Shout moved to Las Vegas where he practiced medicine for the rest of his life. He had charge of the government hospital at Las Vegas Hot Springs, besides attending to a large practice. He traveled many miles by horseback or horse and buggy to visit patients. Shout died on January 18, 1884, having just reached the age of 50 on January 13 of that year. The *Optic* stated that for many years Dr. Shout had been the only physician in Las Vegas and had worked very hard to care for the people for miles around, sometimes traveling hundreds of miles through unsettled country and in all kinds of weather.

One of the most interesting doctors to work at the forts in New Mexico Territory was the courageous Dr. J. M. Whitlock. His full name was John Marmaduke Whitlock and he was Chief Medical Officer at Fort Union. He had a serious conflict with the captain of a company of regulars. The man's name was James "Paddy" Grayson or Grayton or Graydon, depending on which historian is referenced. (For purposes of this story, he will be called Grayson.) Grayson held all "Indians" in contempt, whereas Whitlock viewed Indians as humans to be treated with respect.

According to Dorothy Simpson Beimer, in an article in Spring, 1986 *Old West* magazine, Dr. Whitlock came to New Mexico from

Kentucky in the 1840s, one of the first physicians to arrive to the Las Vegas area. He married Josefita Lucero and they had two children. Kit Carson was a close friend of Whitlock, who had served as surgeon in Carson's regiment of Territorial Militia prior to its re-organization on September 22, 1862. As the Civil War consumed the nation, Whitlock enlisted as surgeon for the First New Mexico Regiment of Volunteers organized at Fort Union.

The diary of a soldier, James Farmer, tells the story of Dr. Whitlock's last hours and his courage in confronting Grayson. The dispute erupted when Whitlock accused Grayson of serious misconduct, asserting that while Grayson was stationed in the Mescalero Apache country with a detachment of soldiers, he had shot down several of them in cold blood. Writing to the editor of a Santa Fe newspaper, Whitlock declared that Grayson and his men were a disgrace to the U.S. Army

That was only the beginning of the conflict. Shortly after he wrote his accusation, Dr. Whitlock went to Fort Stanton in south central New Mexico Territory to ask Colonel Christopher "Kit" Carson to sign a recommendation for his appointment as surgeon with the re-organized militia. Grayson, at the same time, had arrived at Fort Stanton after commanding a massacre on one of his scouting missions. Whitlock had heard that Grayson had surrounded a camp of Mescalero Apaches and ordered his troops to slaughter them all, including women and children.

Dr. Whitlock was furious when he heard of the massacre. It was reported that when Grayson returned from the Indian camp, he was carrying a baby impaled on the bayonet of his rifle and that he had played with the little corpse as though it were a toy animal. Whitlock gave an angry lecture to Grayson, telling him no soldier of the U.S. Army should be guilty of such conduct, punctuating his remarks with some vivid name calling.

Grayson denied improper conduct and demanded that Whitlock take back his statements and that he also retract the accusations that had been sent to the newspaper. Grayson called them "libelous slanderers" and that they reflected on his honor. Whitlock refused. He denounced Grayson fiercely, calling him a murderer and a disgrace to the Army.

Repairs were being made to buildings, so the troops were

housed in tents temporarily. The hospital, too, was housed in a tent for a period of time. On November 8, 1862, while Dr. Whitlock was in the hospital examining patients, Grayson came in and challenged the doctor to a duel.

"I am presently examining and prescribing for my patients," the doctor told Grayson. "As soon as I finish my rounds, I am at your service."

Grayson began to back out of the tent. Then, without warning, he turned and fired at Whitlock. The doctor drew his gun and returned fire. He had nowhere to take cover, and his patients were in danger. Grayson dodged behind the ambulance, still firing. Apparently to draw Grayson's fire away from the patients, the doctor swung after him, exposing himself to Grayson's fire. A bullet from Grayson's gun shattered the butt of Whitlock's pistol and wounded him in the wrist. At the same moment, a bullet from Whitlock's gun struck Grayson near the heart. When the captain fell to the ground, Whitlock threw away his now useless pistol.

When Grayson's company realized their captain was hit, they ran to him. While the doctor knelt over the captain, checking his pulse, the soldiers began firing on him. Their fury mounted when they discovered that their captain was dead.

Again caught off guard, Whitlock turned to the nearest structure for protection--Sutler's Store. He took a shotgun from the gun rack and loaded it. When the soldiers burst through the front door, he hurried toward the back door. Whitlock could confront a lone gunman, but an entire armed company bearing down on him called for a quick retreat. He had almost reached the exit when he was shot in the back and fell dead at the door.

Whitlock's body was thrown into an entrenchment ditch. Soldier after soldier of Grayson's loyal company passed by the body and shot it with revolver, rifle, or shotgun. An examination later revealed that it had been riddled by at least ninety-six gunshot wounds.

By the time the mutilation stopped, the Post was thoroughly alarmed. Assembly was blown and the garrison was ordered to "fall in under arms." The troops surrounded Grayson's company and marched into a hollow square to the parade ground.

Captain Santiago L. Hubbell's Company G, fully armed, was

the first company on the parade ground in response to the long roll. Colonel Kit Carson ordered Grayson's Company H drawn up in front of Company G. He then ordered Company G to "load" and "ready." Company G was ordered to disarm every member of Company H. Colonel Carson stood in anger before them. (No soldier had ever seen Carson in such a towering, threatening rage.)

"I'll have you scoundrels to swing before sunset!" Carson shouted. He indignantly assailed the men for the brutal crime of killing a man who had befriended them all. His fury grew so intense that he had Grayson's men line up and count out. Then he ordered every fourth man to be shot immediately.

But Lieutenant Menhard asked for a brief cooling period. Carson stalked to his tent. Menhard followed him and advised him against any violent act until those who actually were guilty of the atrocity could be brought to justice. Others helped persuade Carson to have the ringleaders in the Whitlock shooting arrested, placed in irons, and held under guard until they could be brought to justice. The men of Company H were confined. Justice failed, however, when three of the soldiers accused of inciting the murder escaped from the

Bernalillo County Jail where they were being held. They then escaped to Mexico. In the end, the cases were dropped.

The humanitarian doctor is remembered as a man who died because he dared to speak up for human rights when such talk was unpopular. Dr. Whitlock was murdered because he defended the right of every law abiding human being to live, regardless of race, creed, gender, or culture.

The doctors continued to ride the trails on horseback or in covered wagons, settling in towns and establishing practices, sometimes engaging in a variety of other endeavors. When the forts were no longer needed, and when the railroad replaced the covered wagons, then small towns began to flourish, and with them, frontier doctors.

REFERENCES

Beimer, Dorothy Simpson, "Pioneer Physicians in Las Vegas, New Mexico: 1880-1911," unpublished manuscript, 1975, in Donnelly Library, New Mexico Highlands University, Las Vegas, New Mexico.

Beimer, Dorothy Simpson. "The Tragic Death of Doctor J. M. Whitlock," *Old West,* Spring, 1986, Vol. 22, No. 3, Whole No. 87, pp. 32,33 - 36-37

Estergreen, M. Morgan. *Kit Carson: A Portrait in Courage.* Norman, Oklahoma: University of Oklahoma Press, 1962, pp. 235-236.

Giese, Dale F. *Forts of New Mexico: Echoes of the Bugle.* Silver City, New Mexico, 1991.

Giese, Dale F., editor. *My Life With the Army in the West: The Memoirs of James E. Farmer, 1858-1898.* Santa Fe, New Mexico: Stagecoach Press, n.d., pp. 48-51.

Hernandez, Mrs. B. C. "A Pioneer Story: The Tragical Death of Doctor J. M. Whitlock in 1868 at Fort Stanton, New Mexico," *New Mexico Historical Review* XVI (January, 1951), pp. 104-105.

Keleher, William A. *Turmoil in New Mexico: 1846-1868.* Santa Fe: The Rydal Press, 1952, pp. 288-291.

Las Vegas Optic, Las Vegas, New Mexico, January 18, 1884.

Lucas, William J. *Why Fort Union?* unpublished manuscript, Las Vegas, New Mexico, n.d. in Donnelly Library, New Mexico Highlands University, Las Vegas, New Mexico.

Simpson, Audrey. "The Fort that Won the West, *New Mexico Magazine,* Vol. 28, No. 12, December, 1950, pp. 14-15.

Twitchell, Ralph Emerson. *The Leading Facts of New Mexican History,* Vol. V., Cedar Rapids: Iowa: The Torch Press, 1917.

CHAPTER 4

The Gunfighters' Doctor

Numerous movies and television shows have depicted Tombstone and its famous characters. From 1955 to 1961, the television series, "The Life and Legend of Wyatt Earp" was popular. It starred Hugh O'Brian as Wyatt Earp, first as U.S. Marshal in Wichita, Kansas, then U. S. Marshal in Dodge City, Kansas; and finally the locale shifted to Tombstone, Arizona for the remainder of the series. The characters often included Bat Masterson and Doc Holliday. Actor Damian O'Flynn played Dr. George Goodfellow in Tombstone, Arizona. In the episode, "Frontier Surgeon," (January 19, 1960) Flynn played a key role as Dr. Goodfellow in an urgent situation to save a man's life.

George Emery Goodfellow, M.D. lived in Tombstone, Arizona in the days of its "wild west" reputation as "the town too tough to die." Goodfellow was born at Downieville, California on December 23, 1855. He was the son of a doctor and mining engineer. He was appointed to Annapolis but was discharged at the age of 17 for fighting. He graduated from Wooster University in Cleveland,

Ohio on February 24, 1876 with his medical degree. He married Katherine Colt of Meadville. He practiced in California and then at Prescott and Fort Lowell in Arizona Territory before moving to Tombstone. He arrived in Tombstone in 1880 at the age of 25. There were twelve "doctors" there, but only he and three others actually had medical degrees. The town had 2,000 residents. Goodfellow hung up his shingle over the Crystal Palace Saloon. When he was not busy removing bullets, Goodfellow, an excellent surgeon, studied other things. He wanted to find a cure for tuberculosis. His background gave him a curiosity and a thirst for knowledge.

The town's newspaper, the *Epitaph,* reflected the violence of the times. The most famous fight was the well-known "gunfight at the O.K. Corral" in which the Earp brothers and "Doc" Holliday met the Clantons for a showdown.

Dr. Goodfellow was not afraid of the many gunfighters who rode into town looking for trouble. Like most of the other men in town, he did not go out on the street without his guns dangling from his gun belt. Some people said he lived a charmed life, often escaping the storms of bullets which often swept the Tombstone streets or saloons like the well-known "Birdcage." The Birdcage Theatre, also called the Birdcage Opera House Saloon, opened its doors on December 25, 1881. It featured a saloon, gambling parlor, theatre and brothel. The many gun fights and knife fights resulted in 26 deaths. There were 140 bullet holes in the ceilings, walls, and floors. The women, known sometimes as "painted ladies," would entertain their customers at very high prices. The Birdcage closed in 1889. Tombstone was a boom town after silver was discovered, and people flocked there to get rich. But when the mines closed, Tombstone receded into history after seven turbulent years.

During those years Dr. Goodfellow had challenges few doctors have ever had. He was brave enough to be the doctor on call for gun slingers and fortune hunters--in one of the west's most violent towns. Not only did Goodfellow care for the town's residents, but he would travel many miles to care for others in surrounding areas. Like most scientists and doctors, he was very observant. He kept notes on his observations. Then he wrote articles for medical journals. He was well known for his expertise in treating gunshot wounds. He wrote several articles in well-known medical journals about the treatment of gunshot wounds. One article was entitled, "Cases of Gunshot Wound of the Abdomen Treated by Operation." Another one explained the doctor's observation that silk often deflects bullets. He wrote, "Note on the Impenetrability of Silk to Bullets." Goodfellow wrote about many things, including an article on the bite of the Gila Monster, a reptile in the Arizona deserts.

Some of the infamous characters in Tombstone gave Dr. Goodfellow plenty of opportunities to try out his ideas in treating gunshot wounds. Wyatt Earp had been Marshall of Dodge City, Kansas and he had experience in dealing with trouble-makers such as cowboys, gamblers, and gunfighters looking for action. When Earp moved to Tombstone, he found that the lively mining town gave him an opportunity to open a business. The Oriental Saloon attracted Wyatt's friends, including Bat Masterson and Luke Short, to work in his new business. Earp was a good friend of Dr. John Henry "Doc" Holliday, a dentist suffering from tuberculosis. "Doc" liked to gamble and didn't mind getting into fights.

Holliday gained his nickname from his practice of dentistry. Born in Griffin, Georgia in 1851, Doc Holliday had developed pulmonary tuberculosis, one of the reasons he traveled to the Southwest in search of a drier climate.

The showdown at the O.K. Corral was a conflict between the two main political groups in town--the Earps and the Clantons. "Old Man" Clanton, or N. H. Clanton, was the boss of a powerful organization. Cattle rustling and robbery were carried on without fear of arrest by the sheriff who was paid off. The Earp brothers--Wyatt, Virgil and Morgan--along with their friend Doc Holliday were in conflict with Tom McLaury, Frank McLaury, Ike Clanton, Billy Clanton and Billy Claiborne. On October 28, 1881, the showdown at the O.K. Corral took place. Thirty rounds were fired in 30 seconds behind the O. K. Corral. Out of 17 shots fired by the Clantons and the McLaurys, there were only three hits at the stable. Yet out of the 17 shots fired by Doc Holliday and the Earps, there were 13 hits. Frank and Tom McLaury, as well as Morgan Earp and Doc Holliday were all wounded, although Virgil and Morgan were not seriously injured and Doc Holliday was barely grazed by a bullet. Tom and Frank McLaury died of their wounds, as did Billy Clanton. (Morgan lived but was killed at a later time.) Ike Clanton, Billy Clairborne and Wes

Fuller were the only cowboys who were not hit, as they ran for their lives. Ike Clanton and John Ringo then left for Mexico.

After the showdown at the O.K. Corral, bystanders took Billy Clanton to Dr. Goodfellow's office where the dying man asked the doctor to take off his boots because he had promised his mother he would never die with his boots on. The doctor carried out the request of the dying man. It was all he could do for him.

One day Virgil Earp was seriously wounded by gunfire as he walked in front of the Eagle Brewery saloon. He then went to the Oriental saloon to tell his brother Wyatt that he was wounded. Wyatt quickly took his brother to the Cosmopolitan Hotel. There Dr. Goodfellow "patched him up." There was one bullet just above the left elbow, causing a fracture of the bone in the arm--the humerus. Virgil Earp also had a back wound where a load of buckshot had hit him. Goodfellow cut away Virgil's shirt, examined the wounds, stopped the bleeding, and then performed surgery. He removed four inches of splintered bone from the elbow and removed the buckshot.

Morgan Earp was shot one night in March of 1882 while playing billiards in Campbell and Hatch's billiard parlor. The shots had exploded through the glass panes of the door which led to an alley. Morgan and George Berry were hit. Wyatt Earp was missed. When Dr. Goodfellow arrived, he discovered a gunshot in Morgan Earp's abdomen. The bullet had passed through his spinal column. Goodfellow was unable to save him. Berry, however, should have lived, as he suffered little more than an abrasion, according the doctor. However, the man died, apparently from shock.

Dr. Goodfellow was used to traveling long distances to help those in need. There was an earthquake in Sonora, Mexico, and the doctor went to help rescue hundreds of injured Mexicans. After that, the Mexicans called him "El Santo Doctor" or "The Doctor Saint." Some made pilgrimages to his home in Tombstone. The Mexican President gave him a horse and a silver double-headed Austrian Eagle which had once belonged to Emperor Maximillian.

One of his longest rides took him, again, into Mexico where his patient was a woman, wife of a rancher, who was giving birth. When a fine son was born, the father, a wealthy rancher, rewarded the doctor with a spring wagon and gold coins.

In July of 1889, Dr. Goodfellow made one of his longest out

of town calls. He rode over 90 miles to Buckskin, Frank Leslie's ranch in Horseshoe canyon. There he found a woman had been shot to death and a man had been badly wounded, victims of their host.

Dr. Goodfellow had a good friend, Dr. John Charles Handy, the leading doctor in Tucson, Arizona. On September 24, 1881, Handy was gunned down and critically wounded. He asked for Goodfellow. The Southern Pacific dispatcher wired for Goodfellow and arranged for trains to speed him to Tucson. Goodfellow was examining the patient by eight p.m., less than six hours after he had received the summons. The bullet had entered the left side of the abdomen and emerged at the tip of the spine, perforating the intestines. At 10:20 p.m., with the help of three Tucson doctors, Goodfellow began repairing eighteen holes in five feet of intestines. At 1:00 a. m., just as he was inserting the last suture, Handy died.

Movies could portray a man like Dr. Goodfellow as a part of the wild west as seen through the eyes of the camera. In real life, Goodfellow saved many lives, and in the end, he gave up his practice in Tombstone to move to Tucson so that he could take over the practice of the friend whose life he had failed to save.

As mentioned before, Las Vegas was one of the early settlements in New Mexico. The west side was established first. Then the "new" town, East Las Vegas, developed east of the Gallinas River as a result of railroad activity when the Railroad came through in 1879. Many businesses were established after that time, mostly on the east side.

One of the men in search of business opportunities was "Doc" Holliday. He was known as a gambler, but he intended to start a business in the booming Las Vegas. According to Las Vegas historian, Marcus Gottschalk, Doc Holliday came to Las Vegas via train in early July, 1879 to cash in on the newly developed east side of town. He immediately acquired a site and solicited the services of contractor W. G. Ward to build a saloon which would be called The Holliday Saloon. It was located on Center Street (now called Lincoln Avenue) in East Las Vegas. The fee totaled $372.50, according to Gattschalk. The little towns which grew up along the railroad line became somewhat lawless frontier towns, often inhabited by men such as buffalo hunters, cowboys and railroad workers. *The Historical Atlas of the Outlaw,* writings by former New Mexico governor Miguel

Otero are cited, listing a total of 29 men killed violently in one month's time in Las Vegas.

On July 26, 1879, an outlaw named Mike Gordon caused trouble. Gordon was a veteran of the Fifth Calvary and had gained a bad reputation, having at his nose bitten off in a gambling quarrel at one time. Gordon was drinking and making threats. Gordon went into a dance hall where his mistress was working. The two began to argue and Gordon began firing gunshots. When one of those entered Holliday's place of business, Holliday fatally shot Gordon in the chest. Holliday's friend, Justice of the Peace H. G. "Hoodoo Brown" Neill dismissed the killing as "excusable homicide." Neill was a friend of Dave "Arkansas" Rudabaugh, the law enforcement offer working for him. Rudabaugh had been in Dodge City, Kansas when Holliday was there. These connections with the law kept Holliday out of jail. Doc had used a shotgun and blew more holes in Gordon than the doctor could count, although the doctor, whose name was not recorded, managed to keep Gordon alive for a while. Gordon died the next day.

A bartender in Las Vegas, Charlie (or Charley) White had also known Doc in Dodge City, Kansas, where they had been fighting before meeting again in Las Vegas. When Holliday learned White was tending bar in Las Vegas, he paid him a visit. White was serving some customers when he recognized his old enemy from Dodge City. White quickly emerged with a gun and the duel began. Holliday fired a shot at White which grazed his head. Holliday thought he had killed the bartender and left the scene. If a doctor attended White--in all probability White did see a physician for his wound--the doctor's name is not known. What is known is that White departed on the next train east to his home in Boston before Holliday had a chance to shoot him again.

While in Las Vegas, Holliday met up with a couple of his more well-known companions, including former lawman Wyatt Earp who spent time in Las Vegas after leaving is job as an officer of the law in Dodge City. Another of Holliday's friends, a former girlfriend, "Big Nose" Kate Elder, met Holliday to rekindle their relationship. Eventually they ended up in Tombstone, Arizona.

Doc Holliday stayed in Las Vegas a little longer but departed after a month or so. Mr. Ward received money from Holliday haphazardly, but when Holliday left town, he still owed Ward $137.50. *Las Vegas Daily Optic* publisher, R. A. Kistler, was cited as saying Las Vegas was simply "too rough" for Holliday.

Holliday, along with Wyatt Earp and other well-known personalities of the time, have been the subjects of numerous popular movies and television shows. Holliday died quietly in Glenwood Springs, Colorado on November 8, 1887 from tuberculosis. He was only 36 years of age.

The "too rough" Las Vegas was a challenge for the physicians and surgeons who lived there. Several accounts given by Miguel Antonio Otero II (October 17, 1859 - August 7, 1944) show how rough New Mexico Territory, particularly Las Vegas, was in the 1800's. Otero was the 16th Governor in the Territory of New Mexico, from 1897 to 1906, and in later life the author of several books. Several of his stories indicate that the doctors in Las Vegas were kept very busy.

A man named Manuel Barela once remarked, looking at a Mr. Romero, "I'll bet fifty dollars I can shoot the third button off that man's vest." The two men were apparently not acquainted. Romero just happened to be in the Barela's line of sight. The outlaw drew his gun and shot Romero through the heart. Police officers arrested him immediately and placed him in the jail behind Charles Ilfeld's store. Barela's family had money and political influence. They hired criminal lawyers to represent Barela. Lawyers postponed his preliminary hearing and it was thought that Barela might go unpunished for the murder.

A few weeks later in new town, a Mr. Beckworth was playing with his pistol, twirled it, showing off. But it discharged and killed a man standing nearby. A crowd gathered around him. Before he was arrested, he protested that the killing was purely accidental. Then he proceeded to demonstrate how the accident had occurred. Again, the pistol discharged, this time killing another bystander, a woman. Beckworth was immediately arrested and placed in the county jail in old town. But Las Vegas had an active Vigilante Committee. That night they broke into the jail and took Beckworth out and hanged him on the infamous windmill of the town. According to Governor Otero's account, they placed a sign on his chest that said, "This is no accident."

Then the vigilantes wondered if they had been fair since they had hanged Beckworth but Barela was still in jail for his murder. It was decided that they should take no chances on a miscarriage of justice, so they returned to the jail, secured Barela and hanged him on the windmill also.

One of the most unusual murders took place at the St. Nicholas Hotel, which was at the corner where the Crockett Building was later built. James Morehead was a well-known traveling salesman. He had stayed up late the night before and did not get up early enough in the morning to eat breakfast at the same time as other patrons of the hotel. He had complained of the surliness and insolence of one of the hotel waiters named Jim Allen. He thought the man might mean trouble. He did not intend to tolerate Allen's attitude. Hence, after sleeping later than usual on March 3, 1880, Morehead entered the dining room of the hotel and seated himself at a table. It was about nine o'clock, just as they were about to close up for breakfast. Allen, the waiter, came up to him and Morehead gave his order, asking for some poached eggs on toast. The waiter told him that he was too late to get eggs and that he would have to take what he could get. Morehead told him he wanted no more of Allen's impudence and abuse, stating that as a guest of the hotel, he was paying for what he got and he insisted on courteous treatment.

Allen started toward the kitchen. Morehead, upset over the confrontation, got up and walked out of the dining room, intending to settle his bill and leave the hotel. As he entered the office, he stopped in front of the water cooler at the end of the counter to get a drink. As he was lifting the glass to his mouth, Allen came rushing into the office from the dining room. He had a cocked pistol in his hand. He called Morehead names and told him to get down on his knees and beg forgiveness or he would be killed.

Morehead made a jump for Allen, and Allen fired one shot. After shooting Morehead, Allen turned and went back into the dining room and closed the door. Morehead was in pain from his wound. He sat down in a chair where his friends found him. He knew he might be dying, and he made a statement as to what had happened. A doctor was not able to save him and he died a few hours later.

The day after the murder, Allen had a preliminary hearing before the District Court. A change of venue was granted to Santa Fe

County. But before a trial took place, Allen and three other prisoners escaped from jail. They were followed by a posse and found near Aguilar Hill, close to the town of Chaperito in San Miguel County. The posse fired upon them without warning and killed all three instantly.

Much of the riotous living centered around a dance hall in Las Vegas--operated by Close and Patterson in a large frame building which was opposite the Castaneda Hotel. The building later burned. In 1870 Sheriff of San Miguel County was Juan Romero. He arrested Jose Ortega and Juan Garcia after they broke into the warehouse of Aniceto Baca in Upper Las Vegas and stole a large quantity of merchandise. Two prisoners were in jail when a group of citizens assembled and took the prisoners from the jail, in spite of the efforts of the sheriff to prevent it. The prisoners were hanged on the hill just west of the present San Miguel County Court House. Such events were fairly rare before the coming of the railroad in 1978. But after that time Las Vegas became a town filled with lawlessness, not quite "too tough to die" as Tombstone, but tough enough. Vicente Silva and his gang were notorious outlaws of the area in the 1890's. Silva murdered his wife, Telesofora Sandoval Silva, in front of his gang, and they were furious. They, in turn, murdered him. It was, indeed, a violent time.

Gunfighters, bounty hunters, and hot-heads were not just the fantasies of movie makers. Such men did exist. The cowboy was a true figure in the culture of the American west, though Hollywood has romanticized that image. The true cowboy led a rough life, often sleeping under the stars after being in the saddle all day. He faced the dangers the cattle and horses often brought in that line of work. Getting thrown from a horse, gored by a steer or a bull, even getting a cut from working on a fence: all those injuries could be serious.

One day a cowpuncher brought his brother to see Dr. F. J. Bancroft at the doctor's house. The doctor examined the leg which had been mangled by gunfire. A crowd had gathered. The doctor operated with an audience. As he sawed through the bone, the brother of the patient pulled out his six-shooter, waved it in the doctor's direction, and threatened that he would kill the doc if his brother died. The doctor calmly continued his work. When he finished the operation and the patient was stable, an onlooker asked him if he had been frightened by the threats. The doctor replied that he, too, had a gun; and he would have been the first to know if death was imminent.

Most frontier doctors carried firearms along with their medical bags. But few had occasion to use the guns. The gunfighters realized they might need the doctor's skills.

REFERENCES

Dunlop, Richard. *Doctors of the American Frontier.* New York: Ballantine Books, 1965.

Hart, Lisa Kay. "Legendary Gambler's Legacy Adds to Town's Colorful History: Holliday in Vegas," La Gente, *Las Vegas Daily Optic,* February 5, 1998, p. 3.

McCarty, Lea F. *The Gunfighters.* Santa Rosa, California: Mike Roberts Color Productions, 1959.

McGrath, Tom. *Vicente Silva and His Forty Thieves: The Vice Criminals of the 80's and 90's.* Las Vegas, New Mexico, 1960.

Otero, Miguel Antonio, *My Life on the Frontier, 1864-1882.* Santa Fe: Sunstone Press, 2007.

CHAPTER 5

Small Town Doctors

Small settlements became villages, villages became towns, and sometimes those towns became cities. The small town doctor, a general practitioner, made house calls and held office hours.

During the late 1950's and the 1960's, the television Western came into its own. Often one of the main characters was a doctor. "Wagon Train," "Rawhide," "Gunsmoke," and "Frontier Doctor" serve as examples.

In "Gunsmoke," the character of "Doc" Adams (Dr. Galen Adams) is an important part of the story, which takes place in Dodge City, Kansas and features U.S. Marshal Matthew "Matt" Dillon (starring James Arness.) The role of Dr. Adams was played by Milburn Stone. He, along with Miss Kitty, played by Amanda Blake, helped make the show popular for twenty years, from 1955 to 1975, the longest-running, prime time, live action drama in the USA--with 635 episodes.

"Frontier Doctor" had a much shorter run but accurately portrayed the life of a doctor in a small western town, Rising Springs, in Arizona Territory. The town's physician, Dr. Bill Baxter (played by actor Rex Allen) is shown riding in a horse-drawn buggy, carrying his black bag to help patients in various situations, often encountering situations that required the use of his gun or his fists to subdue characters such as murdering outlaws.

The role of the doctor traveling west with a wagon train and then settling in a frontier town was portrayed in books, movies and television shows, but those stories were, more often than not, based on true events--real doctors helping in true life situations.

Las Vegas, New Mexico at one time was the largest city in New Mexico Territory. From 1880 to 1911, Las Vegas attracted many health seekers. The climate was conducive to tuberculosis patients seeking sunshine, a high altitude, and a dry atmosphere. The Las Vegas Hot Springs, six miles northwest of Las Vegas, attracted many "consumptives" as well as other health-seekers. By 1900 several sanatoria had been instituted. A few years later the well-known Valmora Industrial Sanatorium was established by Dr. William T. Brown. Valmora is located about 24 miles from Las Vegas and about four miles from Watrous, New Mexico.

Dr. John H. Shout, mentioned in the previous chapter, was one of the early physicians in Las Vegas. In the November 2, 1882 *Las Vegas Daily Optic*, Dr. Shout was referred to as "that humane individual" because of his concern for the destitute and afflicted in the community, a concern which "led him to circulate a subscription paper for their aid." Undoubtedly his concern had arisen because of the many unfortunates arriving in Las Vegas such as George D. Sargent of Riscany Falls, New York. The *Optic* gave an account of the death of the stranger who, on his way to San Francisco, was detained in Las Vegas because of lack of funds and succumbed to his consumption the next day, leaving behind his seven-year-old son. The man was buried at the city's expense. The boy was "penniless and parentless" as described by the *Optic*, but the *Optic* stated that the boy would be provided for by Dr. Shout, if not adopted.

Dr. Shout sometimes was called upon for unpleasant duties. He was requested to witness a legal hanging--of a woman. In 1880 the first woman to be hanged in the Territory was to be executed for murder. Pablita Sandoval had killed Tomas Urbano Baca. They were engaged to be married at Sapello, but she killed her fiancé in a fit of jealous passion and was found guilty of murder in the first degree with the sentence to be hanged.

The county jail was a small one-story adobe building north of the Charles Ilfeld Company's store. There was insufficient space in that location to accommodate the crowds that were expected to attend, and it was decided to conduct the hanging at a tree at Caterina Creek, between the Masonic Cemetery and St. Anthony's Cemetery.

Major Jose D. Sena of Santa Fe had been sent over to read the death warrant. He was the father of Honorable Jose D. Sena, who was for many years Clerk of the Supreme Court of the Territory and later of the State. He delivered an eloquent address to the crowd prior to the execution.

There was a very large crowd to observe the hanging, including many women school children. There was one school in Las Vegas then. It occupied a building on the street north of and parallel to Bridge Street and was conducted by Pablo Maes. There were about forty pupils in all, all boys. The school teacher and his pupils attended to pray and to be taught that crime does not pay.

Professional men were there, including Dr. Shout. Mrs.

Trinidad Romero, whose husband was later Delegate to Congress, was upset when she noticed that the condemned woman's skirt was very thin, worn, and torn. So Mrs. Romero went inside some place and took off her own very fine skirt and sent it over to the "pobrecita," (poor thing) so that she might be hanged decently clad. The Reverend Father Pinard was with the prisoner, giving her spiritual consultation before Sheriff Montoya took over to do his job.

There were two high poles which had probably been intended to be imposing gate posts at the entrance of a small ranch. Sheriff Sacramento Montoya undertook the task of placing a cross beam on the tops of those two poles, constructing his gallows.

The prisoner was riding in a topless prairie schooner drawn by horses. Montoya drove the wagon underneath the cross beam he had placed on the two poles from which a rope had been suspended. He simply reached up, grasped the rope, made a turn of it around the woman's neck, tied a knot in it, and then drove the team and wagon away, leaving her suspended by the neck. But he had failed to bind her hands, so she immediately reached up over her head with both her hands and started to climb the rope, hand over hand. The crowd was astonished and also sympathetic, wanting to release her and send her back to jail with the hope of having her sentence commuted to life imprisonment instead of hanging. But the bungling sheriff was determined to finish the job. He grabbed the prisoner by the legs, dragged her down, unbuckled his pistol belt, pinioned her arms with the belt, and she then slowly strangled. The indignant crowd then turned upon the sheriff, determined to hang him in the same slow way, but they were dissuaded, probably by the doctor and the priest.

People often called a doctor when they were too ill to visit his office, and he would make a house call, even if the home was miles away from his office. The doctor traveling in a light top buggy was often seen, depending on a fast and dependable horse to take him to his patients. Or he might simply ride horseback, carrying his black bag along or taking medicines in a saddle bag. A doctor was often seen walking through the streets of the town to visit a patient in his home, carrying his black bag, the sight of which seemed to bring hope into the hearts of the very ill. But in the 1800's, a doctor's black bag held no magic--only a few key medicines. Besides a few simple items such as his stethoscope, there might be rubbing alcohol to be used for disinfectant or for sponge baths to reduce fever. There was morphine for pain. There was digitalis for the heart. There was quinine for malaria and fever. There was bismuth for stomach ailments. There was castor oil. There were a few tonics and some stimulants such as ammonia. There were tweezers, scissors, various sizes of bandages and gauze pads, and other such items for treating injuries.

In his surgical bag, a doctor might have instruments for emergency surgeries. At his office he used ether or chloroform for surgery. Dr. James Young Simpson discovered the use of chloroform in the 1840s. In 1842 the first physician to use ether as a general anesthetic during surgery was Dr. Crawford Williamson Long. Ether had first been discovered by a Boston dentist, Dr. William T. G. Morton. Both ether and chloroform were used by the time the Civil War broke out in 1861, if and when it was available.

Many small town doctors were over-worked due to the fact that there were few doctors in the area. For instance, Dr. T. A. McKinney of Las Vegas, New Mexico, attempted to serve both East and West Las Vegas (old and new towns). He held office hours on the east side from 7 a.m. to 9 a.m.; on the west side from 9 a.m. to 12 noon; and from 1 p.m. to 8 p.m. on the east side, according to Gladys Thatcher in her study of the early Las Vegas Hospital.

According to the October 3, 1882 *Las Vegas Daily Optic,* Dr. W. J. Pettijohn served as physician to both Hot Springs and Las Vegas. His office was at the Central Drug Store.

Dr. Jacob S. and George S. Easterday, brothers practicing in Albuquerque, New Mexico in the 1890s, worked in town all day and in the country all night.

As cities grew and doctors began to collaborate, it became necessary to establish some rules, so medical societies and medical boards were established. The first meetings of the Las Vegas Medical Society (which later became the New Mexico Medical Society) were held in 1882. Dr. J. H. Shout was President. There was a Board of Medical Examiners at that time, and it approved vaccinating the city population against smallpox, with approval by the City Council. There had been an outbreak of smallpox in that year. On November 19, 1882 the *Las Vegas Optic,* reported that four persons had died at the city hospital. Drs. Peebles, Tipton, Henriquez and Skipworth were to go from house to house and see that everyone was vaccinated. As late as 1889 the physicians were still worried about smallpox. An *Optic* ran an ad that said a man and his wife "who have had smallpox" were wanted to take charge of the City Hospital. They were to apply to Dr. C. C. Gordon, city physician.

Too often a person claimed to be a doctor without having adequate medical training. The Territorial Board of Medical Examiners, located in Las Vegas, was determined to be sure all physicians were qualified. At a July meeting in 1889, a motion was made by Dr. J. M. Cummingham and seconded by Dr. R. H. Longwill of Santa Fe, that the licenses of Dr. A. E. Mintie and Dr. A. C. Stoddard, both of San Francisco, should be revoked, as they had been obtained by fraud.

In the early Territorial period, it was not uncommon for a doctor to travel by buggy or horseback more than a hundred miles to make a call. Dr. Howard Thompson who practiced in Mescalero, New Mexico before moving on to El Paso, Texas, traveled more than 200 miles in one case to attend a rancher's wife having a baby. He went 140 miles in another case to take care of a young man with peritonitis. Trips on horseback of 50 miles or more were common. Dr. L. H. Pate, a general practitioner in Carlsbad, New Mexico, traveled by buggy into ranch country east of town for more than a hundred miles to see a sick patient. The round trip required five days.

Often a physician would treat himself if a remedy was needed and other physicians were unavailable at the time. At the time of the smallpox epidemic in Las Vegas, Dr. J. A. Severson vaccinated himself on his forearm, which later became swollen and painful. But he did not contract smallpox.

Self-medication and surgery were not recommended but were a last resort when a colleague was not available. Dr. F. T. B. Fest of Las Vegas went to extremes, however. Dr. Fest was obese. He decided on a drastic reducing measure, thinking he could operate on himself. Fortunately, he did have two colleagues standing by.

Dr. Fest, having decided to remove superfluous tissue on his abdomen, started the operation on himself in front of a mirror at his office on South Gonzales Street. Under local anesthesia he made his incision. But then he started screaming, "Give me something! Give me something!" Dr. Franklin H. Crail and Dr. H. M. Smith took over the operation and finished it successfully. They removed a piece of flesh forty inches long and four inches wide. Dr. Fest was performing surgery before long, but never again on himself.

Small town doctors may not have been as glamorous as "Doc" Adams on "Gunsmoke" or Dr. Baxter on "Frontier Doctor." But they saved many lives. There were few preventive measures in those days, so infant mortality was high. Immunizations, except for smallpox. were almost unheard of. For those contracting deadly diseases, there were no antibiotics, no cures. A doctor could offer only palliative treatment in many cases. Scarlet fever, cholera, diphtheria, measles whooping cough, typhoid, and many other illness could bring an epidemic to a community. In 1886, tuberculosis accounted for 12 out of 100 deaths in the United States. For years, it was the most prominent cause of death between the ages of 10 and 40, responsible for one third of the deaths of young and middle-aged adults. A doctor without modern medicines was faced with many challenges.

The famous painting, "The Doctor," the 1891 work by Luke Fildes, shows a doctor at the side of a sick child, as the parents look on helplessly. A physician could only do so much, but he could be there, offering as much comfort and assistance as possible.

REFERENCES

Beimer, Dorothy Simpson. *Hovels, Haciendas, and House Calls: The Life of Carl H. Gellenthien, M.D.* Santa Fe: Sunstone Press, 1986.

Beimer, Dorothy Simpson, "Pioneer Physicians in Las Vegas, New Mexico: 1880-1911," unpublished manuscript, 1975, in Donnelly Library, New Mexico Highlands University, Las Vegas, New Mexico.

Las Vegas Daily Optic, Las Vegas, New Mexico, October 3, 1882.

Las Vegas Daily Optic, Las Vegas, New Mexico, January 18, 1884.

Las Vegas Daily Optic, Las Vegas, New Mexico, February 7, 1889.

Las Vegas Daily Optic, Las Vegas, New Mexico, September 11, 1889.

Las Vegas Daily Optic, Las Vegas, New Mexico, January 28, 1911.

Otero, Miguel Antonio, *My Life on the Frontier, 1864-1882.* Santa Fe: Sunstone Press, 2007.

Simpson, Dorothy Audrey. *Audrey of the Mountains: The Story of a Twentieth Century Pioneer Woman.* Santa Fe: Sunstone Press, 2008.

Simpson, Dorothy A. "Doctors of Las Vegas, New Mexico, 1851-1911," in *Las Vegas, New Mexico: 1835-1935.* Compiled and Edited by Edwina Portelle Romero, Published by Friends of the City of Las Vegas Museum and Rough Rider Memorial Collection, Las Vegas, New Mexico, 2018.

Simpson, D.A. *The Cyrenian.* Parker, Colorado: Outskirts Press, 2018, p. 308.

Thatcher, Gladys. *The Origin and Development of the Las Vegas Hospital: 1883 to 1926*, unpublished paper presented to Dr. Lynn I. Perrigo, New Mexico Highlands University, Las Vegas, New Mexico, for Research 550, March 1961, p. 21.

CHAPTER 6

Country Doctors

A country doctor in the frontier west never went anywhere without his two able assistants--his black medical bag and his pistol--one to ward off disease and the other to protect his life.

Dr. Russell Bayly (or Baylay) came to Las Vegas when the railroad came through in 1879. At that time Las Vegas expanded greatly, especially the east side where the railroad tracks and round house were located. Bayly wanted to write a book entitled *Early Days of Las Vegas*. But his schedule kept him so busy he did not find the time.

The January 7, 1882 *Las Vegas Daily Optic* reported that "Doc Bayly's stable was forced open" the night before but his horse was still there. The *Optic* concluded that "Doc is a believer in miracles" but it was generally believed that the thief probably looked at the horse and decided he didn't want it.

Frontier doctors improvised and used anything at hand that could do the job. Some, lacking pain relieving drugs, resorted to the use of liquor. In 1886, Dr. Bayly was "hauled before the County

Commissioners." His crime was that he had prescribed whiskey for an inmate of the county jail. Apparently there if there was a penalty, it was not severe.

Dr. Carl H. Gellenthien became the Director of Valmora Tuberculosis Sanatorium at Valmora, New Mexico, 24 miles north of Las Vegas, about four miles from the village of Watrous. He was the son-in-law of Dr. William T. Brown, a true pioneer doctor who established the TB Sanatorium in the early 1900's. Brown was Gellenthien's mentor when the young doctor completed his medical degree in Chicago and took on the job as Medical Director at Valmora. After Dr. Brown's death on August 30, 1935, Gellenthien took over his job and stayed as the physician at Valmora for the rest of his life.

Dr. Samuel Hassell was a pioneer doctor from Wisconsin, practicing medicine in New Mexico when he met the young doctor Carl Gellenthien who was just out of medical school from Chicago. Dr. Hassell advised the young physician that if he was going to be a country doctor, he had to learn one very important thing: learn to pull teeth. Gellenthien said he hadn't learned how to pull teeth in medical school at the University of Chicago. Hassell told him that if a patient comes to a doctor with a toothache and there is no dentist in the area, it is up to the physician to pull the tooth.

"What if I explain that I'm not a dentist?" Gellenthien retorted.

Then the patient may say, "Well, you're a doctor, ain't you?"

Dr. Hassell advised that any country doctor is expected to take care of all the needs of the people, and that includes dental work if no dentist is available. So young Carl Gellenthien learned to pull teeth after Dr. Hassell gave him the proper dental instruments.

More than once, Dr. Gellenthien had guns pulled on him by hot-heads who wanted revenge for one reason or another, nearly always due to a misunderstanding. Gellenthien carried his own pistol but never had to use it. He was always able to talk his way out of a situation.

Dr. Gellenthien said that a country doctor has to be prepared for anything. A man named Frank from Las Vegas attended a barn dance near wagon Mound and broke his leg. It happened that Dr. Earl Ewert and Dr. Carl Gellenthien were at the dance. Earl had been a classmate of Carl's in Chicago. He became Chief of the Urology

Department of Boston's Lehey Clinic. They put the man by a window and made him comfortable. They had no plaster of Paris in the near-by Wagon Mound Clinic, so Gellenthien sent his nurse to get some regular plaster from one of the merchants in Wagon Mound. The two doctors worked on the leg, wondering why the patient was not complaining of pain. He seemed quite comfortable for a man who had just fractured his tibia. Then they noticed that friends kept passing whiskey up to him through the open window.

The next day Frank went to his regular family doctor in Las Vegas. Dr. H. M. Mortimer, also a graduate of the University of Chicago's medical school. Frank explained what had happened at the dance. The doctor was astonished to see the hard plaster and wondered about it until Frank explained the situation. Mortimer had improvised many times himself, so he understood. He had once set a leg using plaster from a hospital supply that was so old it turned to sand the next day. He had improvised makeshift tools for repairing fractures using nuts, bolts, and even a sacking needle from a local hardware store. He had once used a magazine as a splint to stabilize a fractured arm until he could get the patient to a hospital.

Dr. Henry Hoyt was a physician in Las Vegas, New Mexico and then moved to Bernalillo, New Mexico. He traveled in a buckboard and sent his medicines to his new home by ox train. He, too, had to improvise. Often he would treat a fractured arm or leg with the materials at hand. He had none of the ordinary materials available to use as splints or casts. He would order a panful of adobe mud and use it just as plaster of Paris is used, and he had fine results.

One of Dr. Gellenthien's patients lived in a cave in a canyon wall near Valmora during the Great Depression. The man's wife had died and he was out of work. He had two sons. He had nowhere to go so he made a home out of the cave. With a stove, a cot, and a chair, it became a comfortable place to stay out of the elements. The man often got asthma attacks and would send his 12-year-old son for the doctor at Valmora. Then Gellenthien would make his house call--to the cave. He had to climb half way up the steep canyon wall to reach the cavern where his patient made his abode. The man survived the Depression and was able to find work.

Country doctors visited the rich as well as the poor. People who lived on big ranches, haciendas, or enormous houses in town needed a doctor no less than the poor. Dr. Carl Gellenthien's patients ranged from priests and ministers to associates of the infamous Al Capone. They ranged from famous celebrities such as Greer Garson, Will Rogers, Irvin S. Cobb, Sir Anthony Eden, John L. Lewis, and M.D. Anderson to President Dwight Eisenhower when the doctor was a consultant after the President had a heart attack. Dr. Gellenthien knew many prominent businessmen in all parts of the country. He also belonged to Los Rancheros Visitadores, an exclusive horseback riding group. The annual "trek" near Santa Barbara, California, brought him friendships with great men such as Ronald Reagan and Walt Disney. Although Dr. Gellenthien's patients ranged from the poorest to the rich and famous, he treated them all with the very best he had to offer.

Pioneer doctors such as William T. Brown and Carl H. Gellenthien often performed kitchen table surgery in homes when necessary. Such doctors traveled in all kinds of weather. After the building of railroads, doctors could travel longer distances, not just to see patients but to attend medical meetings. Dr. Gellenthien was traveling by train when an unexpected emergency overtook the travelers. The Grand Canyon Limited pulled out of Dodge City, Kansas with about 200 passengers, heading for Garden City, Kansas. Dr. Gellenthien was headed for home in New Mexico. Somewhere between Dodge City and Garden City, a terrible blizzard began to pile the snow up in heavy drifts and the train could not push through them. It was trapped. There was no communication. When the train failed to show up on time in Garden City, the workers there assumed the train had remained in Dodge City due to the storm. On the other hand, the folks in Dodge City thought the train had reached Garden City.

After a few hours the train ran out of coal so there was no heat. When morning came, food and water ran out. As the second night approached, passengers were desperate. The interior of the train was like a refrigerator as the wind howled at the windows. The doctor did what he could to make people comfortable. People in the Pullman got into bed and covered up. Others put on layers of clothing and wrapped up in blankets. The doctor had his medical bag with him. But nothing could alleviate the discomfort to any great extent. It was nearly 40 hours before the stranded train was discovered. The rescue crew had to break up the train because it was frozen to the track.

There were no serious illnesses. But the Grand Canyon Limited was lucky compared to the Rock Island Express which was to go from Chicago to Kansas City, then to Amarillo, Texas and reach Tucumcari, New Mexico. It was caught in the same snow storm. The passengers on that train burned the passenger's car seats for warmth before they were rescued, and even so, some died of exposure or hypothermia.

Dr. Gellenthien was a railroad surgeon for the Santa Fe Railroad. Rail travel was hazardous in the early days. Injuries were commonplace among the workers. Engineers were often scalded by the steam from the boilers. There were eye injuries from flying cinders. Sometimes limbs or fingers were crushed by the crude coupling devices and had to be amputated. Frequent derailments and collisions resulted in shock and bodily injury. Dr. Gellenthien treated dozens of people each year. His "Discharge from Treatment" records for the Santa Fe Hospital Association indicated a variety of conditions besides common illnesses. Minor injuries included puncture wounds, foreign bodies in the eye, crushed fingers and so on. Sometimes the injuries were much more serious.

On his way to Chicago to an annual scientific meeting of the American Railway Surgeon's Association, Dr. Gellenthien was summoned one morning by the Pullman Conductor, asking the doctor to come with him and see one of the passengers. An elderly woman was lying in her berth dressed in a nightgown. The doctor examined her and then pronounced her dead of an apparent heart attack.

For country doctors as well as their city counterparts, death was the ultimate enemy. As often as a doctor saw death, on the battlefield, in a community epidemic, in a hospital, or in a home, loss of a patient meant a patient's life had ended in spite of all a doctor could do; it was a black mark of "Failure" in the doctor's own thinking.

Television shows that portrayed doctors from small towns accurately depicted their concern for travelers in the surrounding areas, as previously mentioned regarding Dr. Shepherd who visited the wagon train outside of town twice a day during the smallpox epidemic among the travelers who camped outside of town.

In the television series "Rawhide" there were episodes where the cowboys pushing the herd became ill and had to find the nearest town where a doctor's help could be obtained. The series ran from January, 1959 through December, 1965 and starred Eric Fleming as the trail boss, Gil Favor, and Clint Eastwood as Rowdy Yates. "Rawhide" represented the era of the big cattle drives, taking Longhorn cattle from San Antonio, Texas to Sedalia--the true Shawnee Trail, the oldest of the Texas cattle drive routes leading to St. Louis and then to Sedalia and finally to Kansas City as the rails moved west. The series was based on real life experiences recorded in the diary of George C. Duffield who trailed a herd from Texas to Missouri in 1866.

In one episode, "Incident at Red River Station," January 15, 1960, Gil and Rowdy are exposed to smallpox. They find a doctor in a nearby town where smallpox has reached epidemic levels. Dr. Solomon Flood is played by James Dunn. The doctor tries to convince the people to get the smallpox vaccination.

In another episode, Rowdy gets sick and has a rash. After some time a doctor is found. It turns out that Rowdy has cowpox, a much milder illness, than smallpox. Usually anyone who recovered from cowpox would not get smallpox, as the virus built up immunity to the smallpox virus. Early literature portrays the "milk maid" as a beautiful girl. The reason those who worked with cattle were considered good looking is because their faces were not ravaged by the scars of smallpox. They had contracted cowpox at some point and so were immune to smallpox. Many Europeans, and later Americans, were marred with the scars of smallpox until the vaccination was routinely used.

Whether treating patients in towns or the countryside, a physician took his skills where they were needed. The poem, "Frontier Doctor" in *Rawhide Rhymes: Singing Poems of the Old West* by S. Omar Barker, (used with permission) describes the country doctor very well:

> There were cowboys bold in the frontier West,
>   And heroes with flaming guns,
> But of those who served where the long trails curved,
>   They were not the only ones.
> Cowboys, sheriffs, and frontier wives...
>   Add to the list one more
> Whose calling stood for hardihood
>   In those brave days of yore.
>
> A woman hushed a fevered child
>   In a lonely nester's shack,
> While her man rode far by moon and star
>   To fetch the doctor back.
> A cowboy, crushed by a horse's fall,
>   Found pain could be withstood,

Knowing ol' Doc would bust a sock
      To get there if he could.

Few their number and wide the range
      Those frontier doctors rode. . .
A little black bag, a worn-out nag. . .
      To them what debts are owed!
In storm or blizzard, in desert heat,
      For pay or not a cent,
Nothing could block the frontier Doc--
      Whatever the odds, he went!

There were cowboys bold on the old frontier,
      And sheriffs and rangers brave.
Their fame lives yet, but don't forget
      Ol' Doc with a life to save.

REFERENCES

Beimer, Dorothy Simpson. *Hovels, Haciendas, and House Calls: The Life of Carl H. Gellenthien, M.D.* Santa Fe: Sunstone Press, 1986.

Barker, S. Omar, "Frontier Doctor," *Rawhide Rhymes: Singing Poems of the Old West.* Garden City, N.Y.: Doubleday & Company, Inc., 1968.

Las Vegas Daily Optic, Las Vegas, New Mexico, January 7, 1882.

Simpson, Dorothy A. *More About Valmora and Dr. Carl H. Gellenthien, M.D., The Unpublished Chapters, Four of Four: Rancheros y Vaqueros* by Dorothy A. Simpson (formerly Dorothy Simpson Beimer), unpublished manuscript, 2018, Las Vegas, New Mexico, located at the City of Las Vegas Museum and Rough Rider Memorial Collection, Las Vegas, New Mexico.

Thatcher, Gladys. *The Origin and Development of the Las Vegas Hospital: 1883 to 1926*, unpublished paper presented to Dr. Lynn I. Perrigo, New Mexico Highlands University, Las Vegas, New Mexico, for Research 550, March, 1961.

CHAPTER 6

A Missionary Doctor

Dr. Marcus Whitman and his wife Narcissa went to Oregon Territory because they wanted to give the Native Americans medical care and they wanted to convert them to Christianity. Dr. Whitman was the first American doctor in the Northwest, making the trip in 1836. As mentioned before, he was helpful in caring for the sick as he traveled on a wagon train.

When Marcus Whitman was a boy, he had ridden with Dr. Ira Bryant (cousin of poet William Cullen Bryant) to visit the sick. He helped give medicines or set broken bones. In 1825 he studied at the Medical College at Fairfield, New York and then practiced in Pennsylvania, Ontario, and New York.

Whitman was the first graduate of an American medical college to cross the Rocky Mountains to settle in the Oregon Territory. He and Narcissa were married in the Presbyterian Church in Angelica, New York in 1836.

Dr. Whitman built his mission twenty-six miles from the Hudson Bay Company's Fort Walla Walla. Cayuse tribesmen helped him. His mission post was at Waiilatpu, near the present-day Walla Walla. The Whitmans helped the Indians as well as the earliest travelers on the Oregon Trail, assisting the white settlers in the area.

On March 14, 1837, Narcissa gave birth to the first white child to be born in Oregon Territory. They named her Alice Clarissa Whitman.

During the winter of 1842-43 Dr. Whitman rode through blizzards and the threat of Indian attacks over a route which stretched 4,000 miles as far south as Taos and Santa Fe and east through Kansas to Westport, Indiana to try to get help for the Indians. Then he returned over the Oregon Trail with 1,000 settlers on their way to the Willamette Valley. That was also the year he went to Washington, D.C., to try to save the Waiilatpu Mission and to tell the U. S. authorities about the great possibilities of the Pacific Northwest.

Mrs. Whitman not only gave medical assistance to the Native Americans, but she also took in orphaned children from wagon trains. She worked at her husband's side in fighting epidemics of diseases such as cholera, measles, and smallpox. As the Whitmans tried to teach the Native Americans the Christian gospel, they were often misunderstood, sometimes even blamed for the illnesses the Indians suffered.

One day the mountain man Jim Bridger came to Dr. Whitman with a Blackfoot arrowhead in his back. The doctor gave him whiskey for the pain, as there were no alternatives available. Then Bridger bit down on a piece of wood as the doctor's knife dug into the flesh to remove the arrowhead. Other trappers and mountain men came to the doctor to have bullets and arrows removed.

Chief Tilaukait was bitter because two of his sons died of smallpox. When his third son came down with smallpox, the chief was very upset. The Indians treated the boy by first getting him very warm and then dropping him into an icy river. The extreme treatment caused the boy to weaken. Finally he died. The chief blamed the white men for bringing the disease that killed his sons. The Whitmans saw very little progress in their attempts to convert the Indians to Christianity. The Cayuse did not seem interested in the white man's religion.

One Sunday two-year-old Alice was playing outside while her parents were reading. The little girl took two cups with her and said she was going to get some water. A few minutes later a workman told the Whitmans that he had seen two cups floating on the river. At first they thought nothing about it and continued to read. Then suddenly Narcissa realized that something was wrong. It was too quiet. She dropped her book and cried out as she ran through the door and down to the river bank, running up and down the river. An old Cayuse man was fishing in the river. He brought out the body of the small white child.

Dr. Whitman tried artificial respiration on his child, but it was too late. The child was dead. The grieving parents buried the child in a grave near their house. After that, the work seemed ever more difficult. The sad parents found themselves more tired than ever. The doctor still rode on his medical rounds and the couple still prayed for the souls, as well as the bodies, of the Native Americans; but it seemed that the Indians were angry with the white people most of the time.

There was a measles epidemic among the Indians. When the chief's last son died, the Cayuse were furious and bitter. They attacked the doctor, killed him, and then killed Narcissa and the other white people who were at the mission at the time.

Although Dr. Whitman did not succeed in converting many Native Americans while he was alive, his influence had a lasting effect. His dedication and his influence encouraged other white settlers to come to Oregon Territory. Whitman's love for the Cayuse and for all men was evident by the life he had lived, as was that of Narcissa. The doctor and his wife had carried out the Great Commission given by Jesus Christ to go into all the world with the message of the Gospel. (Matthew 28:18-20.) The Whitmans are known as outstanding medical missionaries in the early days of the American West.

The valiant men and women who dared to travel into the unknown frontier should be recognized for their valor. Among those are the doctors who spent their lives dedicated to helping others. They were acquainted with suffering and death. Dr. Carl Gellenthein stated that doctors like himself understood that life and death lay in the Hands of God. The physician was just a willing instrument to try to preserve life as long as possible. Gellenthien quoted The Great Physician, Jesus, Son of God and Son of Man, as He acknowledged the need for doctors when He said: ". . . They that are whole need not a physician; but they that are sick." (This statement was recorded by Luke, a physician, in the Gospel--Luke 5:31.)

A frontier doctor did what he could to preserve life. But when death came, he acknowledged that he had to submit. He faced life and death with the same courage. The frontier west now lies in the pages of history. Dr. Gellenthien of Valmora once said: "We rode hard and we rode long. There was no such word as 'quit.'"

The doctor was in his eighth decade, still practicing medicine when he said, "I will never retire. It's best to die in harness." He worked until he was 89 years of age; he never quit until the Lord called him home. Indeed, he died "in harness." So, too, did Dr. Whitman.

William Shakespeare stated in *Julius Caesar*, Act 2, Scene 2:

Cowards die many times before their deaths,
The valiant never taste of death but once.
Of all the wonders that I yet have heard
It seems to me most strange that men should fear,
Seeing that death, a necessary end,
Will come when it will come.

THE END

REFERENCES

Beimer, Dorothy Simpson. *Hovels, Haciendas, and House Calls: The Life of Carl H. Gellenthien, M.D.* Santa Fe: Sunstone Press, 1986.

Dunlop, Richard Dunlop. *Doctors of the American Frontier*. New York: Ballantine Books, 1965.

Karolevitz, Robert F. *Doctors of the Old West: A Pictorial History of Medicine on the Frontier*. New York: Bonanza Books, MCMLXVII (1967).

Shakespeare, William. "The Tragedy of Julius Caesar," *William Shakespeare, The Complete Works*, Stanley Wells and Gary Taylor, General Editors. Oxford: Clarendon Press, 1988, pp. 609-610.

BIBLIOGRAPHY

Adams, V. K., M.D. "The Medical Pioneers," *New Mexico Magazine,* 28 (May, 1950), pp. 25-37.

Barker, S. Omar, "Frontier Doctor," *Rawhide Rhymes: Singing Poems of the Old West.* Garden City, N.Y.: Doubleday & Company, Inc., 1968.

Beimer, Dorothy Simpson. *Hovels, Haciendas, and House Calls: The Life of Carl H. Gellenthien, M.D.* Santa Fe: Sunstone Press, 1986.

Beimer, Dorothy Simpson, "Pioneer Physicians in Las Vegas, New Mexico: 1880-1911," unpublished manuscript, 1975, in Donnelly Library, New Mexico Highlands University, Las Vegas, New Mexico.

Beimer, Dorothy Simpson. "The Tragic Death of Doctor J. M. Whitlock," *Old West,* Spring, 1986, Vol. 22, No. 3, Whole No. 87, pp. 32,33 - 36-37.

Brooke Bob. "Wagon Tracks West," *Wild West*, August, 1993, pp. 42- 51.

Callon, Milton W. L*as Vegas, New Mexico...The Town that Wouldn't Gamble*. Las Vegas, New Mexico: The Las Vegas Publishing Co, Inc., 1962.

Chávez, Fray Angélico *Origins of New Mexico Families: A Genealogy of the Spanish Colonial Period*. Albuquerque, New Mexico: Museum of New Mexico Press, 1992

Dunlop, Richard Dunlop. *Doctors of the American Frontier*. New York: Ballantine Books, 1965.

Estergreen, M. Morgan. *Kit Carson: A Portrait in Courage.* Norman, Oklahoma: University of Oklahoma Press, 1962, pp. 235-236.

Giese, Dale F. *Forts of New Mexico: Echoes of the Bugle.* Silver City, New Mexico, 1991.

Giese, Dale F., editor. *My Life With the Army in the West: The Memoirs of James E. Farmer, 1858-1898.* Santa Fe, New Mexico: Stagecoach Press, n.d., pp. 48-51.

Guild, Thelma S. and Harvey L. Carter. *Kit Carson: A Pattern for Hero.* Lincoln, Nebraska: University of Nebraska Press, 1984, pp. 226-227.

Hart, Lisa Kay. "Legendary Gambler's Legacy Adds to Town's Colorful History: Holliday in Vegas," La Gente, *Las Vegas Daily Optic,* February 5, 1998, p. 3.

Hernandez, Mrs. B. C. "A Pioneer Story: The Tragical Death of Doctor J. M. Whitlock in 1868 at Fort Stanton, New Mexico," *New Mexico Historical Review* XVI (January, 1951), pp. 104-105.

Hertzler, Arthur E. *The Horse and Buggy Doctor.* New York: Harper & Brothers, 1938.

Karolevitz, Robert F. *Doctors of the Old West: A Pictorial History of Medicine on the Frontier.* New York: Bonanza Books, MCMLXVII (1967).

Keleher, William A. *Turmoil in New Mexico: 1846-1868.* Santa Fe: The Rydal Press, 1952, pp. 288-291.

Las Vegas Daily Optic, Las Vegas, New Mexico, January 7, 1882.

Las Vegas Daily Optic, Las Vegas, New Mexico, October 3, 1882.

Las Vegas Daily Optic, Las Vegas, New Mexico, November 2, 1882.

Las Vegas Daily Optic, Las Vegas, New Mexico, January 18, 1884.

Las Vegas Daily Optic, Las Vegas, New Mexico, February 7, 1889.

Las Vegas Daily Optic, Las Vegas, New Mexico, September 11, 1889.

Las Vegas Daily Optic, Las Vegas, New Mexico, January 28, 1911.

Lewis, Laura H. Shepherd. *My Name is Mary Elizabeth: Westward Through the Eyes of a Child.* X-libris Corporation, 2004.

Lucas, William J. *Why Fort Union?* unpublished manuscript, Las Vegas, New Mexico, 1929, in Donnelly Library, New Mexico Highlands University, Las Vegas, New Mexico.

Otero, Miguel Antonio, *My Life on the Frontier, 1864-1882.* Santa Fe: Sunstone Press, 2007.

McCarty, Lea F. *The Gunfighters.* Santa Rosa, California: Mike Roberts Color Productions, 1959.

McGrath, Tom. *Vicente Silva and His Forty Thieves: The Vice Criminals of the 80's and 90's.* Las Vegas, New Mexico, 1960.

Perrigo, Lynn. *Gateway to Glorieta: A History of Las Vegas, New Mexico.* Boulder, Colorado: Pruett Publishing Company, 1982.

Perrigo, Lynn. *The Rio Grande Adventure: A History of New Mexico.* Chicago: Lyons and Carnaham, 1964.

Shakespeare, William. "The Tragedy of Julius Caesar," *William Shakespeare, The Complete Works*, Stanley Wells and Gary Taylor, General Editors. Oxford: Clarendon Press, 1988, pp. 609-610.

Simpson, Audrey. "The Fort that Won the West, *New Mexico Magazine*, Vol. 28, No. 12, December, 1950, pp. 14-15.

Simpson, D.A. *The Cyrenian.* Parker, Colorado: Outskirts Press, 2018, p. 308.

Simpson, Dorothy Audrey. *Audrey of the Mountains: The Story of a Twentieth Century Pioneer Woman.* Santa Fe: Sunstone Press, 2008.

Simpson, Dorothy A. "Doctors of Las Vegas, New Mexico, 1851-1911," in *Las Vegas, New Mexico: 1835-1935.* Compiled and Edited by Edwina Portelle Romero, Published by Friends of the City of Las Vegas Museum and Rough Rider Memorial Collection, Las Vegas, New Mexico, 2018.

Simpson, Dorothy A. *More About Valmora and Dr. Carl H. Gellenthien, M.D., The Unpublished Chapters, Four of Four: Rancheros y Vaqueros* by Dorothy A. Simpson (formerly Dorothy Simpson Beimer), unpublished manuscript, 2018, Las Vegas, New Mexico, located at the City of Las Vegas Museum and Rough Rider Memorial Collection, Las Vegas, New Mexico.

Struck, " Alvar Núñez Cabeza de Vaca (1490-1564), First European Physician and Surgeon in the United States*," Texas State Journal of Medicine,* 32, 1936, pp. 15-21.

Thatcher, Gladys. *The Origin and Development of the Las Vegas Hospital: 1883 to 1926*, unpublished paper presented to Dr. Lynn I. Perrigo, New Mexico Highlands University, Las Vegas, New Mexico, for Research 550, March, 1961.

Thatcher, Harold F. "Frontier Southwest Americans," unpublished manuscript, Las Vegas, New Mexico, 1978.

The Holy Bible, Containing the Old and New Testaments, Commonly Known as The Authorized (King James) Version, Philadelphia, PA.: The National Bible Press, 1958.

Twitchell, Ralph Emerson. *The Leading Facts of New Mexican History.* Vol. V. Cedar Rapids: Iowa: The Torch Press, 1917.